Fatty Liver Diet Cookbook For Seniors Over 50

Low Carb Recipes And Cleansing Methods To Combat Fatty Liver And Fibrosis

Samantha Bax

Fatty Liver Diet Cookbook For Seniors Over 50
Samantha Bax

Copyright 2023 © Prose Books LLC

Prose Books
Prose Books LLC
Merrimack, NH 03054 USA
email: info@prosebooks.us

Table of Contents

Chapter 1: Introduction

Welcome to "Fatty Liver Cookbook for Seniors Over 50: Low Carb Recipes And Cleansing Methods To Combat Fatty Liver And Fibrosis." Within this cookbook, we have carefully selected a range of recipes tailored specifically to enhance the liver health of individuals aged 50 and above. Our primary aim is to offer a resource for seniors who wish to prioritize their well-being through a nutritious diet.

The liver, being one of the body's organs, plays a role in maintaining our general health. It carries out functions such as detoxifying substances, metabolizing nutrients, regulating cholesterol levels, and producing vital proteins. However, as we age, the liver's functionality may decrease, making it more susceptible to conditions like fatty liver disease.

Fatty liver disease is an increasing concern among seniors, and its prevalence is on the rise. This condition occurs when an excessive amount of accumulates in the liver, hindering its functioning. If left unattended, fatty liver disease can progress into conditions like liver cirrhosis or even liver cancer. However, adopting a diet can significantly improve liver health. Prevent the progression of fatty liver disease.

This cookbook has been thoughtfully crafted as a guide for seniors aiming to optimize their well-being by focusing on their liver health. We have handpicked a selection of recipes that are not only delicious but also incorporate ingredients known for their ability to support liver health. Each recipe has been carefully developed to meet the requirements of seniors over 50, ensuring they receive nutrition while indulging in flavorful meals.

Throughout this cookbook, we will explore a variety of ingredients and cooking techniques that have an impact on liver health. From including fruits and vegetables to incorporating healthy fats and lean proteins, each recipe has been crafted with meticulous attention to detail. We will also delve into the advantages of herbs, spices, and superfoods that have long been recognized for their properties in the liver.

Moreover, we understand that individuals may have restrictions. Therefore, this book offers an array of recipes for preferences such as vegetarian, gluten-free, and dairy-free options. We firmly believe that everyone should have the opportunity to reap the benefits of a diet regardless of their needs.

Within these pages, you will find more than a compilation of recipes. We provide information and expert guidance that goes beyond the basics. Our aim is to offer explanations regarding the advantages each ingredient brings, enabling you to comprehend how they contribute towards promoting liver health.

We will also provide suggestions for planning and preparing meals, making it easier for you to incorporate these recipes into your routine.

It's important to remember that while this cookbook is a resource, it does not replace advice. Suppose you have any existing health conditions or concerns. In that case, it is recommended to consult with your healthcare provider before making significant changes to your diet.

By joining us on this adventure, you're taking a step towards improving the health of your liver. We firmly believe that healthy eating can be both enjoyable and beneficial, and we're thrilled to guide you through this transformative process. Let us come together to embrace a diet that not only excites our taste buds but also nourishes our bodies and enhances our well-being.

In the chapters, you'll discover an assortment of recipes that will inspire you to explore new flavors and textures. Each recipe has been thoughtfully designed with the goal of promoting liver health while satisfying your palate. So put on your apron. Let us embark on this journey together, one mouthwatering recipe at a time!

Chapter 1: Understanding Fatty Liver Disease

Fatty liver disease is a widespread and concerning condition that affects a number of individuals aged 50 and above. It occurs when the liver accumulates an amount of fat, resulting in health complications. In this chapter, we will explore the causes, symptoms, risk factors, and different stages of fatty liver disease.

Additionally, we will emphasize the significance of detection to prevent the progression of the disease into severe conditions such as nonalcoholic steatohepatitis (NASH) fibrosis, and even cirrhosis.

Prevalence among individuals aged 50 and above:

The occurrence of fatty liver disease has been increasingly observed among individuals aged 50 and above. Due to lifestyles, poor dietary choices, and metabolic changes associated with aging, this condition has become a concern for older adults. Research indicates that 25% of individuals in this age group suffer from fatty liver disease. Therefore, it is crucial to raise awareness about this issue and promote detection along with treatment.

Causes, Symptoms, and Risk Factors:

Multiple factors contribute to the development of fatty liver disease. Excessive alcohol consumption is the cause leading to alcoholic fatty liver disease. However, a substantial number of cases are categorized as fatty liver disease (NAFLD), which is not linked to alcohol abuse.

Non-alcoholic fatty liver disease (NAFLD) is often associated with obesity, type 2 diabetes, insulin resistance, metabolic syndrome, high cholesterol levels, and high blood pressure.

The symptoms of fatty liver disease can range from mild to severe. Some individuals may not experience any symptoms at all. Common signs include fatigue, weakness, abdominal discomfort, and weight loss. However, these symptoms can be vague and easily mistaken for conditions. Therefore, undergoing tests is crucial for a diagnosis.

Fatty liver disease is categorized into grades and stages based on the extent of accumulation and liver damage. Grade 1 fatty liver involves buildup with minimal inflammation. Grade 2 fatty liver includes accumulation along with inflammation and cellular damage. These grades are generally reversible through intervention and lifestyle changes.

However, if left untreated, fatty liver disease can progress to stages like non-alcoholic steatohepatitis (NASH), fibrosis (scarring), and eventually cirrhosis. NASH occurs when inflammation and liver cell damage become more pronounced, resulting in the accumulation of tissue. This stage significantly increases the risk of developing cirrhosis—a condition characterized by scarring of the liver tissue, leading to loss of function and potential failure.

The significance of detection cannot be overstated when it comes to managing and preventing the progression of fatty liver disease. It is crucial to undergo health check ups, including liver function tests and imaging studies like ultrasounds or MRIs, as they play a role in detecting the disease at an early stage. Making lifestyle changes such as maintaining a diet, engaging in exercise, losing weight, and refraining from alcohol consumption are essential in effectively managing and reversing fatty liver disease during its initial phases.

In addition to this, timely diagnosis and treatment can help prevent the development of conditions like NASH (alcoholic steatohepatitis), fibrosis, and cirrhosis that pose significant threats to overall health and well-being. By monitoring liver health and seeking attention promptly, we can improve outcomes and prevent long-term complications associated with advanced stages of the disease.

In conclusion, individuals above the age of 50 seniors must have an understanding of fatty liver disease due to its high prevalence and potential complications. Identifying the causes, symptoms, and risk factors associated with this condition empowers people to take measures and seek medical intervention. Prioritizing detection while adopting a lifestyle can help stop the progression of fatty liver disease and safeguard our liver health for a better quality of life.

Chapter 2: The Impact of Diet on Liver Health

The liver, an organ for various metabolic processes, plays a vital role in maintaining overall health and well-being. As we get older, our bodies undergo changes that can significantly impact the health of our liver. One key factor that influences liver function is the food choices we make. In this chapter, we will explore how our diet affects the health of our liver, specifically focusing on individuals aged 50 and above. We will delve into the role that specific ingredients and nutrients play in promoting or improving liver health. Additionally, we will discuss the advantages of following a diet in reducing fat accumulation in the liver and underscore the importance of essential vitamins and minerals for optimal liver function.

Exploring the Impact of Dietary Choices on Liver Health:

Our dietary choices directly affect the well-being of our liver, making it particularly important for individuals over 50 to pay attention to their intake. Consuming a diet high in processed foods, sugar, and unhealthy fats can lead to liver damage. Contribute to non-alcoholic fatty liver disease (NAFLD) development. NAFLD involves a buildup of fat in the liver, which can progress into serious conditions such as cirrhosis or even liver cancer. Therefore, it is crucial to adopt a nutritious diet to maintain liver health.

The Importance of Specific Ingredients and Nutrients in Supporting or Enhancing Liver Health:

Certain ingredients and nutrients have been discovered to promote or enhance the health of the liver. One example is tea, which's rich in antioxidants. Studies indicate that the catechins found in tea can help reduce inflammation, oxidative stress, and fat buildup in the liver, thereby improving its function. Including tea as part of a senior's diet can be beneficial for supporting their liver health.

Furthermore, omega-3 fatty acids found in fish like salmon and mackerel have demonstrated effects on the liver. These fatty acids aid in reducing inflammation and preventing accumulation within the liver, thereby lowering the risk of liver diseases. Seniors should consider incorporating a variety of fish into their diets to benefit from omega-3 fatty acid's positive impact.

The Advantages of a Low-Carbohydrate Diet for Reducing Fat Accumulation in the Liver:

In recent years, there has been increasing popularity surrounding low carbohydrate diets that limit carbohydrate intake while increasing fat and protein consumption. This dietary approach has shown results when it comes to reducing accumulation in the liver. By restricting carbohydrate intake, our bodies are encouraged to utilize stored fat as an energy source, resulting in a decrease in liver fat content.

Seniors who are 50 years old or older can greatly improve their liver health and overall metabolic function by following a diet.

It is important to understand the role of vitamins and minerals in promoting liver function:

Vitamin E, for example, acts as an antioxidant that helps protect liver cells from damage caused by radicals. Additionally, vitamin C plays a role in collagen production, which is vital for maintaining the structural integrity of the liver. Seniors should ensure they meet their recommended intake of these vitamins through a balanced diet or, if necessary, with appropriate supplements.

Moreover, minerals like selenium and zinc are essential for supporting liver health. Selenium acts as an antioxidant and aids in the production of enzymes involved in detoxification processes. On the other hand, zinc contributes to the metabolism of carbohydrates, fats, and proteins, thereby facilitating liver function. Including selenium-rich foods such as Brazil nuts and incorporating sources of zinc like oysters and beef can provide seniors with these minerals to support their liver health.

To conclude this discussion on diet and its impact on liver health among seniors aged 50 or older, making choices significantly influences liver function. Therefore, adopting a nutritious diet becomes paramount for maintaining optimal liver health.

Certain substances and nutrients, such as tea, omega-3 fatty acids, and vital vitamins and minerals, have the potential to enhance or boost liver health. Furthermore, adopting a low carbohydrate diet has demonstrated encouraging outcomes in minimizing the buildup of fat in the liver. By comprehending how our dietary choices affect the well-being of our liver, older individuals can make informed decisions to foster the functioning of this organ.

Chapter 3: The Ultimate Fatty Liver Diet Cookbook

As we get older, it becomes more and more important to prioritize our health and well-being. This is especially true when it comes to taking care of our liver, an organ, for detoxification, metabolism, and overall bodily functions. Seniors over the age of 50 need to be aware of fatty liver disease, a condition where fat accumulates in liver cells and can have consequences. However, with the approach to your diet, you can take charge of your liver health. Enjoy a satisfying and delicious lifestyle.

In this chapter, we are excited to present The Ultimate Fatty Liver Diet Cookbook, specifically created for seniors. We understand that planning and preparing meals can sometimes feel overwhelming, especially when dealing with a health condition like fatty liver disease. That's why we have put care and attention into crafting this cookbook. Each recipe is not only tasty but also nutritionally balanced to support your liver health.

Valuable Tips and Guidelines for Meal Planning and Preparation for Seniors

Before we delve into the mouthwatering recipes, let us share some tips and guidelines for meal planning and preparation.

To get the most out of your journey toward a liver, here are some tips to keep in mind;

Focus on Nutrient-Rich Ingredients:

Each recipe in this cookbook has been thoughtfully chosen to include ingredients that support liver health and provide nutrients. By incorporating these ingredients into your meals, you can nourish your liver. Aid its natural detoxification processes.

Embrace a Low-Carb Lifestyle:

Carbohydrates, ones can burden the liver and worsen fatty liver disease. That's why our recipes emphasize alternatives without compromising taste and satisfaction. This approach helps stabilize blood sugar levels and promotes weight management, both of which are crucial for maintaining a liver.

Practice Portion. Moderation:

While these recipes are designed to be liver-friendly, it's important to consume them in moderation and practice portion control. Obesity and excessive calorie intake are risk factors for fatty liver disease. By being mindful of serving sizes, you can maintain a weight. Reduce strain on your liver.

Now, let us delve into the heart and soul of this cookbook. A collection of recipes specifically designed for seniors over 50 that promote both taste and good liver health.

Our team of experts has carefully curated each recipe to ensure a dining experience while promoting the health of your liver. Whether its breakfast, dinner, snacks, or desserts, we have you covered with a variety of options that cater to every taste preference and occasion.

Start your mornings off with our Rise and Shine Breakfasts. We offer a burst of flavor and nutrients that support liver health. Whether you're craving an omelet packed with vegetables or a satisfying bowl of chia seed pudding, our breakfast recipes provide the perfect balance of nourishment and deliciousness.

For midday meals, our lunch recipes are designed to satisfy and energize you throughout the day. With an array of salads, soups, and protein-rich dishes to choose from, such as grilled chicken salad or lentil soup, we ensure that every bite is both enticing and packed with nutrients.

End your day on a note with our satisfying dinner options. From proteins to vegetables and liver-friendly spices, our recipes showcase an exciting blend of flavors. We aim to provide you with choices that not only satisfy your taste buds but also contribute positively to your liver health.

Are you looking for a healthy dinner option? Whether you're in the mood for salmon or a comforting turkey meatball stew, our collection of dinner recipes has got you covered while also promoting liver health.

Our cookbook offers a range of recipes that incorporate carb-nutrient-rich ingredients specifically chosen to support liver health. Each recipe has been carefully crafted to strike a balance between taste and nutritional benefits. From antioxidant-packed berries to fiber vegetables, these dishes will introduce you to an array of flavors that will complement your liver health journey.

In addition, we provide instructions and nutritional information for every recipe included in this cookbook. These instructions will guide you through each step with confidence, allowing you to easily recreate these dishes in your kitchen. The nutritional information provided gives a breakdown of calories, macronutrients, and other essential details so that you can make informed choices based on your needs.

As you continue reading through this book, we will delve into each recipe individually by providing instructions, nutritional information, and some helpful tips and variations to further enhance your culinary experience. Get ready for a journey that not only promotes the well-being of your liver but also brings delight and contentment to your dining experience.

There's no doubt that the ***Fatty Liver Diet Cookbook For Seniors Over 50*** will transform the way you cook and eat to support liver health. So grab your apron. Prepare yourself for a nourishing adventure towards a healthier liver and a happier you.

Chapter 4: Expert Guidance for Optimal Liver Health

Maintaining a body requires us to prioritize the well-being of our liver, which's an incredibly important organ. This remarkable organ is responsible for functions like detoxification, metabolism, and storing nutrients. Unfortunately, there has been a concerning increase in the occurrence of fatty liver disease in years, posing a threat to public health.

In this chapter, we will explore the insights shared by professionals and experts regarding fatty liver disease. We will also discuss the significance of exercise and physical activity in promoting liver health.

Additionally, we'll provide advice on how to incorporate lifestyle changes that support optimal liver wellness. Lastly, we'll share tips on implementing a fatty liver cleanse to aid in detoxification and promote regeneration of the liver.

<u>Further Insight into Fatty Liver Disease:</u>

To gain an understanding of fatty liver disease, it's crucial to rely on the expertise of professionals and experts who have dedicated their careers to studying this condition. Their knowledge enables us to grasp the causes, symptoms, and potential treatments associated with this disease. Fatty liver disease occurs when fat accumulates abnormally in liver cells, leading to inflammation and potential damage to the organ.

Dr. Sarah Thompson, a known specialist in liver diseases, explains that there are two types of fatty liver disease: alcoholic fatty liver disease (AFLD) and non-alcoholic fatty liver disease (NAFLD).

According to Dr. Thompson, AFLD is directly caused by alcohol consumption. In contrast, NAFLD is associated with metabolic factors like obesity, insulin resistance, and a sedentary lifestyle. Identifying the root causes is crucial for developing treatment plans.

Dr. Michael Rodriguez, a gastroenterologist, stresses the importance of detection through liver function tests and imaging studies to prevent further liver damage and progression to advanced stages of the disease.

Insights on the Significance of Regular Exercise and Physical Activity for Liver Health:

Engaging in exercise and leading a lifestyle have shown positive effects on liver health. Dr. Jessica Patel, an expert in activity and its impact on liver disease, highlights that physical activity helps combat obesity, insulin resistance, and inflammation – all known risk factors for fatty liver disease.

Exercise has been scientifically proven to promote weight loss, reduce content in the liver, and improve insulin sensitivity. Moreover, regular physical activity enhances blood flow to the liver while facilitating its detoxification processes.

Dr. Patel suggests incorporating a mix of exercises like walking or cycling and strength training workouts to enhance liver health. The target is to aim for 150 minutes of moderate-intensity aerobic activity or 75 minutes of vigorous activity each week, along with two or more days dedicated to strength training.

Practical Tips for Embracing Lifestyle Changes that Support Liver Well-being:

Achieving and maintaining a liver involves not only regular exercise but also making lifestyle adjustments. Dr. Jennifer Lopez, a hepatologist specializing in lifestyle interventions for liver health, offers advice for those seeking changes. She advises adopting a nutritious diet that includes plenty of fruits, vegetables, whole grains, lean proteins, and healthy fats. It is important to limit the consumption of added sugars, fats, and processed foods to reduce the risk of fatty liver disease.

Additionally, Dr. Lopez stresses the significance of avoiding alcohol consumption and quitting smoking, as both can significantly harm the liver. She recommends practicing stress management techniques such as meditation, yoga, or deep breathing exercises to alleviate the effects of stress on the liver.

Tips for Incorporating a Cleanse to Promote Liver Detoxification:

Promoting detoxification and supporting liver regeneration can be achieved through a cleanse specifically designed for fatty livers.

While it is important to approach this method and seek guidance from a healthcare professional, Dr. Emily Turner, a doctor, offers some general tips for individuals interested in this approach. She suggests beginning with modifications, which involve cutting out processed foods, alcohol, and added sugars. Instead, focus on consuming foods that are rich in antioxidants, like berries, leafy greens, and cruciferous vegetables.

Dr. Turner also advises incorporating liver herbs and supplements known for their detoxifying properties, such as milk thistle, dandelion root, and turmeric. In addition to these changes, increasing water intake and practicing fasting can further enhance the effectiveness of a fatty liver flush cleanse.

In conclusion, seeking expert guidance is crucial when dealing with fatty liver disease. Healthcare professionals offer insights into the causes, symptoms, and potential treatments for this condition.

Regular exercise is essential for maintaining liver health as it helps combat obesity, insulin resistance, and inflammation. Practical advice on making lifestyle changes like adopting a diet and reducing alcohol consumption is vital in supporting liver wellness.

Finally, suppose you want to support the detoxification process and help your liver regenerate. In that case, it might be worth considering a fatty liver cleanse with the supervision of a healthcare professional. By following their advice, you can take measures to improve your liver health and overall well-being.

Chapter 5: Supportive Measures and Resources

Supporting Measures and Alternative Treatments for Fatty Liver Disease:

Fatty liver disease is a health concern affecting a number of individuals worldwide, especially older adults. While medical intervention plays a role in managing this condition, there are supportive measures and alternative therapies that can greatly contribute to liver health and overall well-being. In this chapter, we will explore ways to support individuals with fatty liver disease, seniors.

Dietary and Lifestyle Adjustments:

One of the methods to promote liver health is through modifications in diet and lifestyle. Seniors with fatty liver disease should focus on adopting a balanced diet of fruits, vegetables, whole grains, and lean proteins. It is crucial to avoid processed foods, high-fat meals, and excessive alcohol consumption. Regular exercise can also aid in weight management. Reduce the risk of complications associated with fatty liver disease.

Alternative Therapies:

Alongside lifestyle changes, several alternative therapies have shown promise in enhancing liver health and combating fatty liver disease. These therapies complement treatments. It can help seniors achieve better outcomes. For example, acupuncture has demonstrated effectiveness in reducing inflammation and improving liver function. Herbal remedies such as milk thistle and dandelion root have also exhibited benefits in promoting liver health.

Before incorporating any therapies into your treatment plan, it's crucial to consult with a healthcare professional.

Exploring the Potential Benefits of Supplements and Vitamins for Liver Health:

While maintaining a diet is essential for liver health, certain supplements and vitamins can offer additional support. However, it's important to remember that these supplements should always be used under the guidance of a healthcare professional. Here are some recommended supplements;

Omega 3 fatty acids: These essential fatty acids possess inflammatory properties that can aid in reducing the accumulation of fat in the liver.

Vitamin E: Renowned for its properties, vitamin E may assist in minimizing liver inflammation and damage caused by radicals.

B complex vitamins: B vitamins play a role in ensuring liver function and may help prevent liver damage.

Further Resources, Websites, and Organizations for Seniors:

If you're dealing with fatty liver disease, it's natural to have questions and seek support. Fortunately, there are resources to help you on your journey towards better liver health. Here are some websites and organizations that can provide seniors with information, educational resources, and support networks;

- **The American Liver Foundation** (www.liverfoundation.org) is an organization dedicated to promoting liver health. Their website offers articles, patient resources, and support groups.

- **The National Institute of Diabetes and Digestive and Kidney Diseases** (www.niddk.nih.gov) provides information on liver diseases, including liver disease. You can find details about treatment options and research updates on their website.

- **MedlinePlus** (www.medlineplus.gov) is a trusted resource for health information. They have a range of articles and fact sheets on liver diseases, diets, and treatment options.

- **LiverSupport.com** (www.liversupport.com) is another website that offers various articles, recipes, and lifestyle tips for individuals looking to improve their liver health.

Additionally, it's beneficial for seniors to connect with support groups or clinics specializing in liver diseases. These groups can provide information, resources, and a supportive community.

Furthermore, it's essential for seniors to regularly monitor their liver health. Routine check ups, blood tests, and imaging studies can help track the progression of fatty liver disease and identify any signs of worsening conditions.

Maintaining communication with healthcare professionals who can provide guidance and recommend interventions is extremely important.

Knowing When to Seek Medical Assistance:

Throughout the journey of managing fatty liver disease, seniors must be aware of when they should seek assistance. If they experience pain, jaundice (yellowing of the skin or eyes), persistent fatigue, or any other concerning symptoms, they should promptly consult their healthcare provider. Taking action can often prevent complications and ensure timely treatment.

To sum up, by incorporating measures exploring therapies and utilizing available resources, seniors can actively promote liver health and effectively manage fatty liver disease. With adjustments to diet and lifestyle, potential benefits from supplements and vitamins, access to websites and organizations for information, and regular monitoring of liver health, seniors can improve their overall well-being while effectively addressing this condition.

Chapter 6 – Breakfast Recipes

Welcome to Chapter 6 of our ***Fatty Liver Diet Cookbook for Seniors Over 50***. Starting your day with breakfast is a way to energize yourself and provide essential nutrients. In this chapter, we have carefully selected seven breakfast recipes specifically designed for seniors who are concerned about maintaining a healthy liver.

Each recipe in this chapter has been thoughtfully crafted to promote liver well-being without compromising on taste. We understand the significance of beginning your day with meals that are both delicious and mindful of your health.

Our breakfast recipes incorporate ingredients that are beneficial for individuals dealing with fatty liver disease. You will discover a variety of options that are high in fiber and saturated fats and packed with vitamins and antioxidants. Whether you prefer an omelet, a comforting bowl of oatmeal, a protein-rich wrap, or a delightful parfait, we have something for everyone.

These recipes did not offer simplicity in preparation. Also, allows you to customize them according to your personal preferences. We have included vegetables, fruits, whole grains, lean proteins, and heart-healthy fats to ensure that your breakfast aligns with your liver health goals.

Don't forget having a nutritious breakfast is important to kickstart your day on a note. By incorporating these breakfast recipes into your routine, you're taking a proactive approach to improving your liver health and overall well-being. Start your mornings with nourishing dishes that will keep you satisfied and energized throughout the day.

Now, let us explore these mouthwatering breakfast recipes specially designed to support seniors like yourself in their journey toward better liver health. From scrambled eggs to delightful chia seed pudding, there's something for everyone. So, let us embark together on this healthy breakfast adventure!

Recipe 1: Scrambled Egg and Spinach Breakfast Wrap

Prep Time: 10 minutes - Cooking Time: 10 minutes - Number of Servings: 2

Ingredients:

- 4 large eggs
- 1 cup fresh spinach, chopped
- 1/4 cup diced red bell pepper
- 2 whole wheat tortillas
- 1/4 cup low-fat shredded cheddar cheese
- Salt and pepper to taste
- Cooking spray

Cooking Instructions:

1. In a bowl, whisk the eggs and season with a pinch of salt and pepper.
2. Heat a non-stick skillet over medium heat and lightly coat it with cooking spray.
3. Add the diced red bell pepper and cook for 2 minutes until slightly softened.
4. Add the chopped spinach to the skillet and cook for an additional 2 minutes until wilted.
5. Pour the beaten eggs into the skillet and gently scramble them with the vegetables until fully cooked.
6. Warm the whole wheat tortillas in a dry skillet or microwave.
7. Divide the scrambled egg mixture between the tortillas, sprinkle with shredded cheddar cheese, and fold them into wraps.

Nutrition Values (per serving):

- - Calories: 275 kcal
- - Protein: 17g
- - Carbohydrates: 17g

Note: This protein-packed breakfast wrap is a quick and healthy way to start your day. The spinach adds vitamins and minerals, making it a great choice for seniors concerned about their liver health.

Recipe 2: Oatmeal with Berries and Almonds

Prep Time: 5 minutes - Cooking Time: 10 minutes - Number of Servings: 2

Ingredients:

- 1 cup old-fashioned oats
- 2 cups unsweetened almond milk
- 1/2 cup mixed berries (blueberries, strawberries, raspberries)
- 2 tablespoons sliced almonds
- 1 tablespoon honey (optional)
- 1/2 teaspoon ground cinnamon
- A pinch of salt

Cooking Instructions:

1. In a saucepan, combine the old-fashioned oats and almond milk. Add a pinch of salt and bring to a gentle boil.
2. Reduce the heat to low and simmer for about 5-7 minutes, stirring occasionally, until the oats are tender and the mixture thickens.
3. Remove from heat and stir in the ground cinnamon.
4. Divide the oatmeal between two bowls.
5. Top with mixed berries and sliced almonds. Drizzle with honey if desired.

Nutrition Values (per serving):

- - Calories: 275 kcal
- - Protein: 8g
- - Fiber: 8g

Note: This oatmeal breakfast is rich in fiber and antioxidants from the berries, making it a heart-healthy choice for seniors. Adjust sweetness to taste by adding honey or your preferred sweetener.

Recipe 3: Greek Yogurt Parfait with Walnuts and Honey

Prep Time: 5 minutes - Cooking Time: 0 minutes - Number of Servings: 2

Ingredients:

- 2 cups non-fat Greek yogurt
- 1/2 cup chopped walnuts
- 1/4 cup fresh blueberries
- 1/4 cup sliced bananas
- 2 tablespoons honey (optional)
- 1/2 teaspoon vanilla extract

Instructions:

1. In two serving glasses or bowls, layer the Greek yogurt, chopped walnuts, fresh blueberries, and sliced bananas.
2. Drizzle a teaspoon of honey (if desired) over each parfait.
3. Sprinkle a dash of vanilla extract over the top for added flavor.

Nutrition Values (per serving):

- - Calories: 320 kcal
- - Protein: 20g
- - Fiber: 3g

Note: This yogurt parfait is high in protein and provides healthy fats from walnuts, making it a satisfying and liver-friendly breakfast option for seniors with fatty liver disease. Adjust sweetness with honey according to preference.

Recipe 4: Veggie and Cheese Omelet

Prep Time: 10 minutes - Cooking Time: 10 minutes - Number of Servings: 2

Ingredients:

- 4 large eggs
- 1/2 cup diced bell peppers (red, green, or yellow)
- 1/4 cup diced onions
- 1/4 cup diced tomatoes
- 1/4 cup low-fat shredded cheddar cheese
- 1 tablespoon olive oil
- Salt and pepper to taste
- Chopped fresh herbs (e.g., parsley or chives) for garnish (optional)

Cooking Instructions:

1. In a bowl, whisk the eggs and season with a pinch of salt and pepper.
2. Heat olive oil in a non-stick skillet over medium heat.
3. Add diced bell peppers and onions to the skillet and sauté for 3-4 minutes until they start to soften.
4. Add diced tomatoes and cook for an additional 2 minutes.
5. Pour the beaten eggs over the vegetables in the skillet and cook until the edges set.
6. Sprinkle the shredded cheddar cheese evenly over one-half of the omelet.
7. Carefully fold the omelet in half with a spatula.
8. Cook for another 2-3 minutes until the cheese melts and the omelet is fully cooked.
9. Garnish with fresh herbs if desired before serving.

Nutrition Values (per serving):

- - Calories: 235 kcal
- - Protein: 14g
- - Carbohydrates: 6g

Note: This vegetable and cheese omelet is a great source of protein and essential vitamins. It's a satisfying breakfast option for seniors with fatty liver disease. You can customize the vegetables to your preference.

Recipe 5: Banana and Walnut Breakfast Muffins

Prep Time: 15 minutes - Cooking Time: 20 minutes - Number of Servings: 12 muffins

Ingredients:

- 2 ripe bananas, mashed
- 1/2 cup unsweetened applesauce
- 1/4 cup honey or maple syrup
- 2 large eggs
- 1 teaspoon vanilla extract
- 1 1/2 cups whole wheat flour
- 1 teaspoon baking powder
- 1/2 teaspoon baking soda
- 1/2 teaspoon ground cinnamon
- 1/4 teaspoon salt
- 1/2 cup chopped walnuts

Cooking Instructions:

1. Preheat your oven to 350°F (175°C). Grease a muffin tin or use muffin liners.

2. In a mixing bowl, combine the mashed bananas, applesauce, honey or maple syrup, eggs, and vanilla extract. Mix well.

3. In another bowl, whisk together the whole wheat flour, baking powder, baking soda, ground cinnamon, and salt.

4. Gradually add the dry ingredients to the wet ingredients and mix until just combined. Do not overmix.

5. Gently fold in the chopped walnuts.

6. Spoon the batter into the muffin tin, filling each cup about 2/3 full.

7. Bake for 18-20 minutes, or until a toothpick inserted into a muffin comes out clean.

8. Allow the muffins to cool for a few minutes in the tin before transferring them to a wire rack to cool completely.

Nutrition Values (per muffin):

- - Calories: 150 kcal
- - Protein: 3g
- - Fiber: 2g

Note: These banana and walnut breakfast muffins are a delightful and fiber-rich morning treat for seniors with fatty liver disease. The whole wheat flour and walnuts add a wholesome touch.

Recipe 6: Chia Seed Pudding with Mixed Berries

Prep Time: 5 minutes (plus overnight refrigeration) - Cooking Time: 0 minutes - Number of Servings: 2

Ingredients:

- 1/4 cup chia seeds
- 1 cup unsweetened almond milk
- 1/2 teaspoon vanilla extract
- 1 tablespoon honey (optional)
- 1/2 cup mixed berries (blueberries, strawberries, raspberries)
- Sliced almonds or shredded coconut for garnish (optional)

Instructions:

1. In a bowl, combine chia seeds, almond milk, vanilla extract, and honey (if desired). Stir well.

2. Cover the bowl and refrigerate it overnight or for at least 4 hours to allow the chia seeds to absorb the liquid and create a pudding-like consistency.

3. Before serving, give the mixture a good stir to evenly distribute the chia seeds.

4. Divide the chia seed pudding into two serving glasses or bowls.

5. Top with mixed berries and garnish with sliced almonds or shredded coconut if desired.

Nutrition Values (per serving):

- - Calories: 180 kcal

- - Protein: 4g

- - Fiber: 10g

Note: Chia seed pudding is a nutrient-rich, high-fiber breakfast that's easy to prepare. The mixed berries add antioxidants, while chia seeds offer omega-3 fatty acids. It's a perfect option for seniors with fatty liver disease.

Recipe 7: Spinach and Mushroom Breakfast Quesadilla

Prep Time: 15 minutes - Cooking Time: 10 minutes - Number of Servings: 2

Ingredients:

- 4 large whole wheat tortillas
- 1 cup fresh spinach leaves
- 1 cup sliced mushrooms
- 1/2 cup diced red bell pepper
- 1/2 cup shredded low-fat mozzarella cheese
- 4 large eggs
- Salt and pepper to taste
- Cooking spray

Instructions:

1. In a bowl, whisk the eggs and season with a pinch of salt and pepper.

2. Heat a non-stick skillet over medium heat and lightly coat it with cooking spray.

3. Add sliced mushrooms and diced red bell pepper to the skillet. Sauté for 3-4 minutes until the vegetables soften.

4. Push the vegetables to one side of the skillet and pour the beaten eggs into the other side. Scramble the eggs until fully cooked.

5. Lay out the whole wheat tortillas and divide the cooked eggs, sautéed vegetables, fresh spinach leaves, and shredded mozzarella cheese evenly between two tortillas.

6. Top each with another tortilla to create quesadillas.

7. Heat a clean skillet or griddle over medium-high heat and lightly coat it with cooking spray.

8. Cook each quesadilla for 2-3 minutes on each side or until the tortillas are crispy and the cheese is melted.

9. Remove from heat and let them cool for a minute before slicing into wedges.

Nutrition Values (per serving):

- - Calories: 340 kcal
- - Protein: 21g
- - Carbohydrates: 29g

Note: This spinach and mushroom breakfast quesadilla is a satisfying and savory option for breakfast.

Chapter 7 – Lunch Recipes

Welcome to Chapter 7 of our *Fatty Liver Diet Cookbook for Seniors Over 50*. This chapter is about liver-friendly lunch recipes. Lunchtime is an opportunity to nourish your body with a meal that supports your liver health and overall well-being.

In this chapter, we've carefully curated seven lunch recipes specifically tailored for seniors dealing with fatty liver disease. We understand the importance of a satisfying lunch in managing your liver health and keeping you energized throughout the day.

Each recipe in this chapter focuses on incorporating ingredients known to promote liver health, such as proteins, fiber-rich vegetables, whole grains, and healthy fats. Our aim is to make these recipes not only delicious but easy to prepare, making them perfect for seniors looking to maintain a diet that's kind to their liver.

From salads to comforting soups and flavorful wraps, our lunch recipes offer options that cater to different tastes and dietary needs. Whether you prefer something refreshing or a substantial dish, you'll find something here that will satisfy your appetite.

By choosing these recipes, you're taking a step towards improving your liver health. These meals are not designed to support your liver but also provide a dining experience.

By taking each bite, you're not providing nourishment to your body. Also aiding your liver in its quest for optimal health.

So, let us embark on an adventure together as we explore these mouthwatering lunch recipes. We can make lunchtime a nutritious experience that contributes to the well-being of your liver and overall vitality.

Whether you indulge in a grilled chicken salad or savor a comforting bowl of soup, rest assured that you're making choices that promote the health of your liver and enhance your vitality.

Recipe 8: Grilled Chicken and Vegetable Salad

Prep Time: 15 minutes - Cooking Time: 15 minutes - Number of Servings: 2

Ingredients:

- 2 boneless, skinless chicken breasts
- 2 cups mixed salad greens (e.g., spinach, arugula, and romaine)
- 1 cup cherry tomatoes, halved
- 1/2 cucumber, sliced
- 1/4 red onion, thinly sliced
- 1/4 cup crumbled feta cheese
- 2 tablespoons balsamic vinaigrette dressing
- Olive oil for grilling
- Salt and pepper to taste

Cooking Instructions:

1. Preheat your grill or grill pan to medium-high heat.
2. Brush the chicken breasts with a little olive oil and season with salt and pepper.
3. Grill the chicken for about 6-7 minutes per side or until cooked through and no longer pink in the center.
4. Remove the chicken from the grill and let it rest for a few minutes before slicing it into strips.
5. In a large bowl, combine the salad greens, cherry tomatoes, cucumber, and red onion.
6. Add the sliced chicken on top of the salad.
7. Sprinkle with crumbled feta cheese and drizzle with balsamic vinaigrette dressing.
8. Toss the salad gently to combine all the ingredients.

Nutrition Values (per serving):

- - Calories: 320 kcal
- - Protein: 35g
- - Fiber: 4g

Note: This grilled chicken and vegetable salad is a protein-packed lunch option that's light on the liver. It's loaded with colorful vegetables and healthy fats from the dressing and feta cheese.

Recipe 9: Quinoa and Black Bean Salad

Prep Time: 15 minutes - Cooking Time: 15 minutes (for quinoa) - Number of Servings: 4

Ingredients:

- 1 cup quinoa, rinsed and drained
- 2 cups water
- 1 can (15 ounces) black beans, drained and rinsed
- 1 cup corn kernels (fresh, frozen, or canned)
- 1 red bell pepper, diced
- 1/2 red onion, finely chopped
- 1/4 cup fresh cilantro, chopped
- Juice of 2 limes
- 2 tablespoons olive oil
- 1 teaspoon ground cumin
- Salt and pepper to taste
- Avocado slices for garnish (optional)

Cooking Instructions:

1. In a medium saucepan, combine the rinsed quinoa and water. Bring to a boil, then reduce the heat to low, cover, and simmer for 15 minutes or until the quinoa is tender and the water is absorbed. Fluff with a fork and let it cool.
2. In a large bowl, combine the cooked quinoa, black beans, corn, diced red bell pepper, and chopped red onion.
3. In a small bowl, whisk together the lime juice, olive oil, ground cumin, salt, and pepper to make the dressing.
4. Pour the dressing over the quinoa mixture and toss to coat all the ingredients evenly.
5. Sprinkle the chopped cilantro on top and gently toss again.
6. Chill in the refrigerator for at least 30 minutes before serving.
7. Garnish with avocado slices, if desired, before serving.

Nutrition Values (per serving):

- - Calories: 300 kcal
- - Protein: 10g
- - Fiber: 9g

Note: This quinoa and black bean salad is a fantastic lunch option for seniors with fatty liver disease. It's packed with plant-based protein, fiber, and a variety of colorful vegetables, making it both delicious and supportive of liver health.

Recipe 10: Baked Salmon with Lemon-Dill Sauce

Prep Time: 10 minutes - Cooking Time: 20 minutes - Number of Servings: 2

Ingredients:

- 2 salmon fillets (68 ounces each)
- 1 lemon, thinly sliced
- 2 tablespoons fresh dill, chopped
- 1 clove garlic, minced
- 2 tablespoons olive oil
- Salt and pepper to taste
- For the LemonDill Sauce:
- 1/4 cup Greek yogurt
- 1 tablespoon fresh lemon juice
- 1 teaspoon fresh dill, chopped
- Salt and pepper to taste

Cooking Instructions:

1. Preheat your oven to 375°F (190°C). Line a baking sheet with parchment paper.
2. Place the salmon fillets on the prepared baking sheet.
3. Season the salmon with minced garlic, salt, and pepper.
4. Arrange lemon slices on top of each fillet and sprinkle with fresh dill.
5. Drizzle olive oil evenly over the salmon.
6. Bake in the preheated oven for about 15-20 minutes or until the salmon flakes easily with a fork.
7. While the salmon is baking, prepare the Lemon-Dill Sauce by mixing Greek yogurt, lemon juice, chopped dill, salt, and pepper in a small bowl.
8. Once the salmon is done, serve it with a dollop of Lemon-Dill Sauce on top.

Nutrition Values (per serving):

- - Calories: 350 kcal
- - Protein: 30g
- - Omega-3 Fatty Acids: 1,500mg

Note: This baked salmon with Lemon-Dill Sauce is a protein-rich lunch option that's rich in heart-healthy omega-3 fatty acids. It's a flavorful and nutritious choice for seniors with fatty liver disease.

Recipe 11: Turkey and Avocado Wrap

Prep Time: 10 minutes - Cooking Time: 0 minutes - Number of Servings: 2

Ingredients:

- 4 whole wheat tortillas
- 8 slices lean turkey breast
- 1 ripe avocado, sliced
- 1 cup mixed greens (e.g., spinach, arugula, and lettuce)
- 1/2 cup cherry tomatoes, halved
- 2 tablespoons Greek yogurt
- 1 tablespoon Dijon mustard
- Salt and pepper to taste

Assembly Instructions:

1. Lay out the whole wheat tortillas on a clean surface.
2. Spread 1/2 tablespoon of Greek yogurt on each tortilla.
3. Spread 1/2 tablespoon of Dijon mustard on top of the Greek yogurt on each tortilla.
4. Place 2 slices of lean turkey breast on each tortilla.
5. Layer avocado slices, mixed greens, and cherry tomatoes on top of the turkey.
6. Season with a pinch of salt and pepper.
7. Roll up each tortilla tightly, securing the contents.
8. Slice each wrap in half and serve.

Nutrition Values (per serving):

- - Calories: 320 kcal
- - Protein: 20g
- - Fiber: 8g

Note: This turkey and avocado wrap is a balanced and satisfying lunch option for seniors with fatty liver disease. It combines lean protein, healthy fats from avocado, and a variety of vegetables for a flavorful and nutritious meal.

Recipe 12: Lentil and Vegetable Soup

Prep Time: 15 minutes - Cooking Time: 30 minutes - Number of Servings: 4

Ingredients:

- 1 cup dried green or brown lentils, rinsed and drained
- 1 onion, finely chopped
- 2 carrots, diced
- 2 celery stalks, diced
- 2 cloves garlic, minced
- 1 can (14 ounces) diced tomatoes
- 6 cups low-sodium vegetable broth
- 1 teaspoon ground cumin
- 1/2 teaspoon smoked paprika
- Salt and pepper to taste
- Fresh parsley for garnish (optional)

Cooking Instructions:

1. In a large pot, heat a bit of olive oil over medium heat.
2. Add chopped onions, diced carrots, and diced celery. Sauté for about 5 minutes until they start to soften.
3. Add minced garlic, ground cumin, smoked paprika, salt, and pepper. Cook for another minute until fragrant.
4. Add rinsed lentils, diced tomatoes, and vegetable broth to the pot.
5. Bring the mixture to a boil, then reduce the heat to low, cover, and simmer for about 20-25 minutes or until the lentils and vegetables are tender.
6. Taste and adjust the seasoning as needed.
7. Serve the soup hot, garnished with fresh parsley if desired.

Nutrition Values (per serving):

- - Calories: 250 kcal
- - Protein: 13g
- - Fiber: 10g

Note: This lentil and vegetable soup is a wholesome and fiber-rich lunch option for seniors with fatty liver disease. Lentils are an excellent source of plant-based protein and fiber, making this soup both satisfying and supportive of liver health.

Recipe 13: Caprese Salad with Grilled Chicken

Prep Time: 15 minutes - Cooking Time: 15 minutes - Number of Servings: 2

Ingredients:

- 2 boneless, skinless chicken breasts
- 2 cups cherry tomatoes, halved
- 1 cup fresh mozzarella cheese balls (bocconcini), halved
- 1/4 cup fresh basil leaves
- 2 tablespoons balsamic glaze
- 2 tablespoons extra-virgin olive oil
- Salt and pepper to taste

Cooking Instructions:

1. Preheat your grill or grill pan to medium-high heat.
2. Season the chicken breasts with a drizzle of olive oil, salt, and pepper.
3. Grill the chicken for about 6-7 minutes per side or until cooked through and no longer pink in the center.
4. Remove the chicken from the grill and let it rest for a few minutes before slicing it into thin strips.
5. In a large bowl, combine the halved cherry tomatoes, halved mozzarella cheese balls, and fresh basil leaves.
6. Drizzle with extra-virgin olive oil and balsamic glaze.
7. Season with a pinch of salt and pepper.
8. Toss the salad gently to combine.
9. Top the salad with the sliced grilled chicken.

Nutrition Values (per serving):

- - Calories: 400 kcal
- - Protein: 35g
- - Calcium: 400mg

Note: This Caprese salad with grilled chicken is a protein-packed and calcium-rich lunch option that's also low in saturated fats. It combines the flavors of fresh tomatoes, mozzarella, and basil with grilled chicken for a satisfying and liver-friendly meal.

Recipe 14: Whole Wheat Pasta with Pesto and Cherry Tomatoes

Prep Time: 15 minutes - Cooking Time: 15 minutes - Number of Servings: 4

Ingredients:

- 8 ounces whole wheat pasta (penne or spaghetti)
- 2 cups cherry tomatoes, halved
- 1/2 cup fresh basil leaves
- 1/4 cup grated Parmesan cheese
- 1/4 cup pine nuts, toasted
- 2 cloves garlic, minced
- 1/4 cup extra-virgin olive oil
- Salt and pepper to taste
- Lemon wedges for garnish (optional)

Cooking Instructions:

1. Cook the whole wheat pasta according to the package instructions until al dente. Drain and set aside.
2. In a food processor, combine the fresh basil leaves, grated Parmesan cheese, toasted pine nuts, minced garlic, and a pinch of salt and pepper.
3. Pulse the mixture while slowly drizzling in the extra-virgin olive oil until you achieve a smooth pesto sauce.
4. In a large bowl, toss the cooked pasta with the cherry tomato halves and the prepared pesto sauce until well coated.
5. Season with additional salt and pepper to taste.
6. Garnish with lemon wedges if desired before serving.

Nutrition Values (per serving):

- - Calories: 380 kcal
- - Protein: 12g
- - Fiber: 6g

Note: This whole wheat pasta with pesto and cherry tomatoes is a flavorful and fiber-rich lunch option for seniors with fatty liver disease. It's a balance of whole grains, healthy fats from pine nuts and olive oil, and the freshness of cherry tomatoes and basil.

Chapter 8: Main Course Recipes

Welcome to Chapter 8 of our ***Fatty Liver Diet Cookbook for Seniors Over 50***, dedicated to promoting a liver. In this section, we're excited to present a selection of course recipes that are not only delicious but also beneficial for your liver.

We understand the importance of maintaining a diet that supports liver health while still providing enjoyment. Each recipe in this chapter has been carefully chosen with seniors in mind, focusing on combating fatty liver disease without compromising on taste.

Our main course recipes have been thoughtfully crafted to incorporate proteins, whole grains, fiber-rich vegetables, and healthy fats. All elements of a liver-friendly diet. Whether you crave succulent fish, tender chicken, or hearty vegetarian options, we offer a variety of choices to satisfy your palate.

These recipes did not nurture your liver. Also, provide wholesome and satisfying meals. We firmly believe that eating well should be an experience. With these course recipes, you can relish your meals while proactively supporting liver health.

Alright, let us dive into these delicious main course recipes. From salmon dishes to satisfying quinoa bowls, each recipe is designed with your liver's health in focus. Prepare yourself to enjoy the flavors and take a stride toward a happier version of yourself.

Recipe 15: Lemon Herb Baked Salmon

Prep Time: 10 minutes - Cooking Time: 20 minutes - Number of Servings: 2

Ingredients:

- 2 salmon fillets (68 ounces each)
- Zest of 1 lemon
- Juice of 1 lemon
- 2 cloves garlic, minced
- 2 tablespoons fresh parsley, chopped
- 1 tablespoon fresh dill, chopped
- 1 tablespoon olive oil
- Salt and pepper to taste
- Lemon wedges for garnish (optional)

Cooking Instructions:

1. Preheat your oven to 375°F (190°C). Line a baking sheet with parchment paper.

2. In a small bowl, combine the lemon zest, lemon juice, minced garlic, fresh parsley, fresh dill, olive oil, salt, and pepper to make a marinade.

3. Place the salmon fillets on the prepared baking sheet.

4. Brush the salmon fillets with the prepared lemon herb marinade, ensuring they are well coated.

5. Bake in the preheated oven for about 15-20 minutes or until the salmon flakes easily with a fork.

6. Remove the salmon from the oven and let it rest for a few minutes before serving.

7. Garnish with lemon wedges if desired.

Nutrition Values (per serving):

- - Calories: 320 kcal
- - Protein: 34g
- - Omega-3 Fatty Acids: 1,200mg

Note: This lemon herb baked salmon is a flavorful and heart-healthy main course. Salmon is rich in omega-3 fatty acids, which can benefit liver health. The zesty lemon and fresh herbs add a burst of flavor to this nutritious dish.

Recipe 16: Mediterranean Chickpea Salad

Prep Time: 15 minutes - Cooking Time: 0 minutes - Number of Servings: 4

Ingredients:

- 2 cans (15 ounces each) chickpeas, drained and rinsed
- 1 cucumber, diced
- 1 cup cherry tomatoes, halved
- 1/2 red onion, finely chopped
- 1/4 cup Kalamata olives, pitted and sliced
- 1/4 cup fresh parsley, chopped
- 1/4 cup fresh mint leaves, chopped
- 1/4 cup crumbled feta cheese (optional)
- 2 tablespoons extra-virgin olive oil
- Juice of 1 lemon
- 2 cloves garlic, minced
- Salt and pepper to taste

Assembly Instructions:

1. In a large mixing bowl, combine the chickpeas, diced cucumber, halved cherry tomatoes, finely chopped red onion, sliced Kalamata olives, fresh parsley, and fresh mint leaves.

2. If using, sprinkle crumbled feta cheese on top.

3. In a small bowl, whisk together the extra-virgin olive oil, lemon juice, minced garlic, salt, and pepper to make the dressing.

4. Drizzle the dressing over the salad and toss gently to combine all the ingredients.

5. Taste and adjust the seasoning as needed.

6. Serve immediately or refrigerate for later. It's even more flavorful when chilled.

Nutrition Values (per serving):

- - Calories: 290 kcal
- - Protein: 11g
- - Fiber: 10g

Note: This Mediterranean chickpea salad is a protein-rich, fiber-packed main course. It's loaded with plant-based protein from chickpeas and a variety of colorful vegetables, making it a satisfying and liver-friendly meal.

Recipe 17: Grilled Lemon Herb Chicken

Prep Time: 10 minutes - Cooking Time: 15 minutes - Number of Servings: 2

Ingredients:

- 2 boneless, skinless chicken breasts
- Zest of 1 lemon
- Juice of 1 lemon
- 2 cloves garlic, minced
- 2 tablespoons fresh thyme leaves
- 1 tablespoon fresh rosemary, chopped
- 1 tablespoon olive oil
- Salt and pepper to taste
- Lemon wedges for garnish (optional)

Cooking Instructions:

1. Preheat your grill or grill pan to medium-high heat.
2. In a small bowl, combine the lemon zest, lemon juice, minced garlic, fresh thyme leaves, fresh rosemary, olive oil, salt, and pepper to make a marinade.
3. Season the chicken breasts with a drizzle of olive oil, salt, and pepper.
4. Brush the chicken breasts with the prepared lemon herb marinade, ensuring they are well coated.
5. Grill the chicken for about 6-7 minutes per side or until cooked through and no longer pink in the center.
6. Remove the chicken from the grill and let it rest for a few minutes before serving.
7. Garnish with lemon wedges if desired.

Nutrition Values (per serving):

- - Calories: 280 kcal
- - Protein: 40g
- - Vitamin C: 30mg

Note: This grilled lemon herb chicken is a mouthwatering and protein-rich main course option. The combination of lemon and fresh herbs adds a burst of flavor to the tender chicken breasts, making it a delightful choice for liver health-conscious seniors.

Recipe 18: Vegetable Stir-Fry with Tofu

Prep Time: 15 minutes - Cooking Time: 15 minutes - Number of Servings: 4

Ingredients:

- 14 ounces firm tofu, cubed
- 2 tablespoons low-sodium soy sauce
- 1 tablespoon sesame oil
- 1 tablespoon rice vinegar
- 1 tablespoon honey or maple syrup
- 2 tablespoons vegetable oil
- 2 cloves garlic, minced
- 1 teaspoon fresh ginger, minced
- 1 red bell pepper, sliced
- 1 yellow bell pepper, sliced
- 1 cup broccoli florets
- 1 cup snap peas
- 1 carrot, julienned
- 2 cups cooked brown rice
- Sesame seeds for garnish (optional)
- Sliced green onions for garnish (optional)

Cooking Instructions:

1. In a small bowl, mix together the low-sodium soy sauce, sesame oil, rice vinegar, and honey (or maple syrup) to create the stir-fry sauce.

2. Heat 1 tablespoon of vegetable oil in a large wok or skillet over medium-high heat.

3. Add the cubed tofu and stir-fry for about 3-4 minutes until it's lightly browned. Remove the tofu from the skillet and set it aside.

4. In the same skillet, add the remaining tablespoon of vegetable oil. Add minced garlic and ginger, and stir-fry for about 30 seconds until fragrant.

5. Add the sliced red and yellow bell peppers, broccoli florets, snap peas, and julienned carrot. Stir-fry for about 5-7 minutes until the vegetables are tender-crisp.

6. Return the cooked tofu to the skillet and pour the stir-fry sauce over the tofu and vegetables. Stir to coat everything evenly.

7. Serve the vegetable stir-fry over cooked brown rice.

8. Garnish with sesame seeds and sliced green onions if desired.

Nutrition Values (per serving, including brown rice):

- - Calories: 350 kcal

- - Protein: 15g

- - Fiber: 7g

Recipe 19: Baked Chicken and Vegetable Medley

Prep Time: 15 minutes - Cooking Time: 25 minutes - Number of Servings: 2

Ingredients:

- 2 boneless, skinless chicken breasts
- 2 cups mixed vegetables (e.g., broccoli, carrots, and bell peppers), cut into bite-sized pieces
- 1 tablespoon olive oil
- 1 teaspoon dried thyme
- 1 teaspoon dried rosemary
- 2 cloves garlic, minced
- Salt and pepper to taste
- Lemon wedges for garnish (optional)

Cooking Instructions:

1. Preheat your oven to 375°F (190°C). Line a baking sheet with parchment paper.
2. Place the chicken breasts on one-half of the prepared baking sheet.
3. In a mixing bowl, combine the mixed vegetables, olive oil, dried thyme, dried rosemary, minced garlic, salt, and pepper. Toss to coat the vegetables evenly.
4. Spread the seasoned vegetables on the other half of the baking sheet.
5. Bake in the preheated oven for about 20-25 minutes, or until the chicken is cooked through and the vegetables are tender.
6. Remove from the oven and let it rest for a few minutes.
7. Garnish with lemon wedges if desired before serving.

Nutrition Values (per serving):

- - Calories: 320 kcal
- - Protein: 40g
- - Fiber: 5g

Note: This baked chicken and vegetable medley is a well-rounded main course option. It combines lean protein from chicken with a variety of colorful vegetables, creating a balanced and liver-friendly meal.

Recipe 20: Spaghetti Squash Primavera

Prep Time: 15 minutes - Cooking Time: 45 minutes - Number of Servings: 4

Ingredients:

- 1 medium-sized spaghetti squash
- 2 tablespoons olive oil
- 1 onion, finely chopped
- 2 cloves garlic, minced
- 1 cup cherry tomatoes, halved
- 1 cup broccoli florets
- 1 cup bell peppers (mix of red and yellow), thinly sliced
- 1 cup baby spinach leaves
- 1/4 cup grated Parmesan cheese (optional)
- Salt and pepper to taste
- Fresh basil leaves for garnish (optional)

Cooking Instructions:

1. Preheat your oven to 375°F (190°C).
2. Cut the spaghetti squash in half lengthwise and scoop out the seeds. Place the squash halves, cut side down, on a baking sheet lined with parchment paper.
3. Roast the spaghetti squash in the preheated oven for about 40-45 minutes, or until the flesh is tender and easily shreds with a fork. Let it cool slightly.
4. Using a fork, scrape the flesh of the spaghetti squash to create "noodles" and set them aside.
5. In a large skillet, heat olive oil over medium heat. Add the chopped onion and minced garlic, sautéing until fragrant, and the onion is translucent.
6. Add the halved cherry tomatoes, broccoli florets, and sliced bell peppers to the skillet. Cook for about 5-7 minutes until the vegetables are tender-crisp.
7. Stir in the baby spinach leaves and cook for an additional 2-3 minutes until wilted.
8. Toss the cooked spaghetti squash "noodles" into the skillet with the sautéed vegetables. Mix well.
9. Season with salt and pepper to taste.
10. If desired, sprinkle grated Parmesan cheese on top and garnish with fresh basil leaves before serving.

Nutrition Values (per serving, without Parmesan cheese):

- - Calories: 120 kcal
- - Protein: 2g
- - Fiber: 4g

Recipe 21: Baked Cod with Lemon-Dill Sauce

Prep Time: 10 minutes - Cooking Time: 20 minutes - Number of Servings: 2

Ingredients:

- 2 cod fillets (68 ounces each)
- Zest of 1 lemon
- Juice of 1 lemon
- 2 tablespoons fresh dill, chopped
- 1 clove garlic, minced
- 2 tablespoons olive oil
- Salt and pepper to taste
- Lemon wedges for garnish (optional)

Cooking Instructions:

1. Preheat your oven to 375°F (190°C). Line a baking sheet with parchment paper.
2. Place the cod fillets on the prepared baking sheet.
3. In a small bowl, combine the lemon zest, lemon juice, minced garlic, fresh dill, olive oil, salt, and pepper to make a marinade.
4. Brush the cod fillets with the prepared lemon-dill marinade, ensuring they are well coated.
5. Bake in the preheated oven for about 15-20 minutes or until the cod flakes easily with a fork.
6. Remove the cod from the oven and let it rest for a few minutes before serving.
7. Garnish with lemon wedges if desired.

Nutrition Values (per serving):

- - Calories: 260 kcal
- - Protein: 30g
- - Vitamin C: 30mg

Note: This baked cod with lemon-dill sauce is a light and protein-rich main course option that's gentle on the liver. The combination of lemon and dill adds a burst of flavor to the tender and flaky cod fillets.

Chapter 9 – Sides Recipes

Welcome to Chapter 9 of our *Fatty Liver Diet Cookbook for Seniors Over 50* where we delve into a selection of side dishes that perfectly complement your liver meals. While the main courses often steal the spotlight, a chosen side dish can truly enhance your dining experience. Provide essential nutrients to support your liver's health.

In this chapter, we have curated seven versatile side dish recipes that are not only mouthwatering but also specifically designed to promote liver well-being. These sides are carefully crafted with ingredients focusing on vegetables, grains, and legumes to boost your overall nutrition.

Our goal is to take you on a journey that prioritizes the health of your liver with every meal. Whether you're in the mood for a salad, a comforting grain-based side dish, or an innovative vegetable medley, you'll find an array of options perfectly tailored to complement your courses.

These recipes are ideal for seniors who actively manage fatty liver disease. They offer both nourishment and flavor, ensuring that you can savor a satisfying meal while taking positive steps towards better liver health.

So, let us embark on this exploration of side dishes:

Each recipe in this collection provides a blend of flavors and textures, from roasted vegetables to satisfying quinoa salads. These dishes did not nourish your body. Also, bring joy to your meals. Embark on a journey towards a liver with every bite.

Recipe 22: Roasted Asparagus with Lemon and Parmesan

Prep Time: 10 minutes - Cooking Time: 15 minutes - Number of Servings: 4

Ingredients:

- 1 bunch of asparagus spears, tough ends trimmed
- 2 tablespoons olive oil
- Zest of 1 lemon
- Juice of 1 lemon
- 1/4 cup grated Parmesan cheese
- Salt and pepper to taste
- Lemon wedges for garnish (optional)

Cooking Instructions:

1. Preheat your oven to 425°F (220°C).
2. Place the trimmed asparagus spears on a baking sheet.
3. Drizzle olive oil over the asparagus and toss to coat them evenly.
4. Sprinkle lemon zest and juice over the asparagus.
5. Season with salt and pepper to taste.
6. Roast in the preheated oven for about 12-15 minutes or until the asparagus is tender and slightly crispy.
7. Remove from the oven and sprinkle grated Parmesan cheese over the hot asparagus.
8. Garnish with lemon wedges if desired before serving.

Nutrition Values (per serving):

- - Calories: 80 kcal
- - Protein: 4g
- - Fiber: 2g

Note: This roasted asparagus with lemon and Parmesan is a simple yet flavorful side dish that pairs perfectly with your main courses. Asparagus is rich in folate and antioxidants, making it a nutritious addition to your liver-friendly diet.

Recipe 23: Quinoa and Vegetable Pilaf

Prep Time: 15 minutes - Cooking Time: 25 minutes - Number of Servings: 4

Ingredients:

- 1 cup quinoa, rinsed and drained
- 2 cups low-sodium vegetable broth
- 1 tablespoon olive oil
- 1 onion, finely chopped
- 2 cloves garlic, minced
- 1 red bell pepper, diced
- 1 yellow bell pepper, diced
- 1 zucchini, diced
- 1 cup frozen peas
- 1 teaspoon ground cumin
- Salt and pepper to taste
- Fresh parsley for garnish (optional)

Cooking Instructions:

1. In a medium saucepan, combine the quinoa and low-sodium vegetable broth. Bring to a boil, then reduce the heat to low, cover, and simmer for about 15-20 minutes, or until the quinoa is cooked and the liquid is absorbed. Remove from heat and let it sit, covered, for 5 minutes. Fluff with a fork.

2. In a large skillet, heat olive oil over medium heat. Add the chopped onion and sauté until translucent.

3. Add minced garlic, diced red bell pepper, diced yellow bell pepper, and diced zucchini to the skillet. Sauté for about 5 minutes until the vegetables are tender-crisp.

4. Stir in the frozen peas, ground cumin, salt, and pepper. Cook for an additional 2-3 minutes until the peas are heated through.

5. Add the cooked quinoa to the skillet with the sautéed vegetables. Toss everything together until well combined.

6. Taste and adjust the seasoning as needed.

7. Garnish with fresh parsley if desired before serving.

Nutrition Values (per serving):

- - Calories: 280 kcal
- - Protein: 8g
- - Fiber: 6g

Note: This quinoa and vegetable pilaf is a wholesome and fiber-rich side dish that pairs well with a variety of main courses.

Recipe 24: Roasted Brussels Sprouts with Balsamic Glaze

Prep Time: 10 minutes - Cooking Time: 25 minutes - Number of Servings: 4

Ingredients:

- 1 pound Brussels sprouts, trimmed and halved
- 2 tablespoons olive oil
- Salt and pepper to taste
- 2 tablespoons balsamic glaze
- 1/4 cup chopped toasted pecans (optional)

Cooking Instructions:

1. Preheat your oven to 400°F (200°C).
2. Place the halved Brussels sprouts on a baking sheet.
3. Drizzle olive oil over the Brussels sprouts and toss to coat them evenly.
4. Season with salt and pepper to taste.
5. Roast in the preheated oven for about 20-25 minutes, or until the Brussels sprouts are tender and slightly crispy, stirring once halfway through.
6. Remove from the oven and drizzle with balsamic glaze.
7. If desired, sprinkle chopped toasted pecans over the Brussels sprouts before serving.

Nutrition Values (per serving, without pecans):

- - Calories: 90 kcal
- - Protein: 3g
- - Fiber: 3g

Note: These roasted Brussels sprouts with balsamic glaze are a flavorful and nutrient-packed side dish. Brussels sprouts are rich in fiber, vitamins, and antioxidants, making them a healthy addition to your liver-friendly diet.

Recipe 25: Garlic Mashed Cauliflower

Prep Time: 10 minutes - Cooking Time: 15 minutes - Number of Servings: 4

Ingredients:

- 1 large head of cauliflower, cut into florets
- 2 cloves garlic, minced
- 2 tablespoons unsalted butter or olive oil
- 1/4 cup low-fat Greek yogurt
- Salt and pepper to taste
- Chopped fresh chives for garnish (optional)

Cooking Instructions:

1. Steam or boil the cauliflower florets until they are tender, about 10-12 minutes.
2. Drain the cooked cauliflower and transfer it to a large bowl.
3. In a small saucepan, melt the unsalted butter (or heat the olive oil) over low heat. Add minced garlic and sauté for about 1-2 minutes until fragrant. Be careful not to brown the garlic.
4. Add the garlic-butter (or garlic-olive oil) mixture and low-fat Greek yogurt to the bowl with the cooked cauliflower.
5. Use a potato masher or a hand blender to mash the cauliflower until smooth and creamy.
6. Season with salt and pepper to taste.
7. If desired, garnish with chopped fresh chives before serving.

Nutrition Values (per serving):

- - Calories: 70 kcal
- - Protein: 3g
- - Fiber: 3g

Note: This garlic-mashed cauliflower is a nutritious and lower-carb alternative to traditional mashed potatoes. It's a delicious side dish that complements a variety of main courses while providing the benefits of cauliflower, which is rich in vitamins and fiber.

Recipe 26: Cucumber and Tomato Salad

Prep Time: 10 minutes - Cooking Time: 0 minutes - Number of Servings: 4

Ingredients:

- 2 cucumbers, sliced
- 2 large tomatoes, diced
- 1/2 red onion, thinly sliced
- 1/4 cup fresh dill, chopped
- 2 tablespoons extra-virgin olive oil
- 2 tablespoons red wine vinegar
- Salt and pepper to taste
- Feta cheese crumbles for garnish (optional)

Assembly Instructions:

1. In a large mixing bowl, combine the sliced cucumbers, diced tomatoes, thinly sliced red onion, and chopped fresh dill.
2. In a small bowl, whisk together the extra-virgin olive oil and red wine vinegar to make the dressing.
3. Drizzle the dressing over the cucumber and tomato mixture.
4. Season with salt and pepper to taste.
5. Toss the salad gently to combine all the ingredients.
6. If desired, sprinkle feta cheese crumbles on top before serving.

Nutrition Values (per serving, without feta cheese):

- - Calories: 90 kcal
- - Protein: 2g
- - Fiber: 2g

Note: This cucumber and tomato salad is a refreshing and hydrating side dish that's perfect for seniors with fatty liver disease. It's a simple yet flavorful way to enjoy the goodness of fresh vegetables and herbs.

Recipe 27: Sweet Potato and Quinoa Salad

Prep Time: 15 minutes - Cooking Time: 20 minutes - Number of Servings: 4

Ingredients:

- 1 cup quinoa, rinsed and drained
- 2 cups water or low-sodium vegetable broth
- 2 medium sweet potatoes, peeled and diced
- 2 tablespoons olive oil
- 1 teaspoon smoked paprika
- 1/2 teaspoon cumin
- Salt and pepper to taste
- 1/4 cup chopped fresh cilantro
- 1/4 cup dried cranberries
- 1/4 cup chopped pecans
- Juice of 1 lemon

Cooking Instructions:

1. In a medium saucepan, combine the quinoa and water (or vegetable broth). Bring to a boil, then reduce the heat to low, cover, and simmer for about 15-20 minutes, or until the quinoa is cooked and the liquid is absorbed. Remove from heat and let it sit, covered, for 5 minutes. Fluff with a fork.

2. Preheat your oven to 400°F (200°C).

3. In a large bowl, toss the diced sweet potatoes with olive oil, smoked paprika, cumin, salt, and pepper until they are evenly coated.

4. Spread the seasoned sweet potatoes on a baking sheet and roast in the preheated oven for about 15-20 minutes or until they are tender and slightly caramelized.

5. In a serving bowl, combine the cooked quinoa, roasted sweet potatoes, chopped fresh cilantro, dried cranberries, and chopped pecans.

6. Drizzle the lemon juice over the salad and toss gently to combine all the ingredients.

7. Season with additional salt and pepper to taste if needed.

Nutrition Values (per serving):

- - Calories: 320 kcal
- - Protein: 6g
- - Fiber: 7g

Note: This sweet potato and quinoa salad is a delightful combination of flavors and textures. It's a nutrient-rich side dish that's packed with fiber, vitamins, and a touch of natural sweetness from sweet potatoes and cranberries.

Recipe 28: Garlic Lemon Broccoli

Prep Time: 10 minutes - Cooking Time: 10 minutes - Number of Servings: 4

Ingredients:

- 1 pound broccoli florets
- 3 cloves garlic, minced
- 2 tablespoons olive oil
- Zest of 1 lemon
- Juice of 1 lemon
- Salt and pepper to taste
- Grated Parmesan cheese for garnish (optional)

Cooking Instructions:

1. Steam the broccoli florets for about 3-4 minutes or until they are bright green and tender-crisp. Drain and set aside.
2. In a large skillet, heat olive oil over medium heat. Add minced garlic and sauté for about 1-2 minutes until fragrant.
3. Add the steamed broccoli to the skillet and toss to coat with the garlic-infused olive oil.
4. Drizzle lemon zest and lemon juice over the broccoli.
5. Season with salt and pepper to taste.
6. Sauté for an additional 2-3 minutes until the broccoli is heated through and well coated.
7. If desired, sprinkle grated Parmesan cheese on top before serving.

Nutrition Values (per serving, without Parmesan cheese):

- - Calories: 90 kcal
- - Protein: 3g
- - Fiber: 3g

Note: This garlic lemon broccoli is a zesty and nutritious side dish that pairs well with various main courses. Broccoli is rich in fiber and vitamins, and the addition of lemon and garlic adds delightful flavor.

Chapter 10 – Snack Recipes

Welcome to Chapter 10 of our ***Fatty Liver Diet Cookbook for Seniors Over 50***, where we dive into a collection of wholesome and satisfying snacks that are designed to support the health of your liver. Snacking doesn't have to be something you feel guilty about; it can be an opportunity to nourish your body with options that are also good for you.

In this chapter, we have put together seven snack recipes specifically tailored to the needs of seniors managing fatty liver disease. These snacks did not taste great. Also, it provides essential nutrients while still being enjoyable.

We understand the importance of snacking, and our recipes are created to help you regulate your blood sugar levels. Make healthier choices for the well-being of your liver. Whether you're in the mood for something sweet or a dip, we have a variety of options that will satisfy your cravings.

Our snack recipes focus on using foods, lean proteins, and heart-healthy fats so you can indulge in snacks without compromising your liver health goals. It's time to elevate snacking from an afterthought to a part of your balanced diet.

Join us on this journey as we explore mouthwatering snacks that are perfect for seniors managing fatty liver disease. These snacks demonstrate the concept that you can indulge in treats while simultaneously promoting a liver.

Recipe 29: Greek Yogurt and Berry Parfait

Prep Time: 10 minutes - Number of Servings: 2

Ingredients:

- 1 cup low-fat Greek yogurt
- 1 cup mixed berries (e.g., strawberries, blueberries, raspberries)
- 2 tablespoons honey
- 1/4 cup granola (choose a low-sugar option)
- 1/4 teaspoon cinnamon (optional)

Assembly Instructions:

1. In two serving glasses or bowls, start by adding a layer of low-fat Greek yogurt to the bottom.
2. Add a layer of mixed berries on top of the yogurt.
3. Drizzle 1 tablespoon of honey over each parfait.
4. Sprinkle granola evenly over the berries and yogurt.
5. If desired, dust a pinch of cinnamon over the top for added flavor.
6. Serve immediately or refrigerate for a cool and refreshing snack.

Nutrition Values (per serving):

- - Calories: 230 kcal
- - Protein: 12g
- - Fiber: 4g

Note: This Greek yogurt and berry parfait is a delightful and protein-rich snack that's gentle on the liver. Greek yogurt provides probiotics and protein, while berries offer antioxidants and fiber, making it a nutritious option for seniors with fatty liver disease.

Recipe 30: Hummus and Veggie Snack Platter

Prep Time: 10 minutes - Number of Servings: 2

Ingredients:

- 1/2 cup hummus (storebought or homemade)
- Baby carrots
- Cucumber slices
- Cherry tomatoes
- Bell pepper strips (red, yellow, or green)
- Celery sticks

Assembly Instructions:

1. Arrange a variety of fresh vegetables, such as baby carrots, cucumber slices, cherry tomatoes, bell pepper strips, and celery sticks, on a serving platter.
2. Place a bowl of hummus in the center of the platter.
3. Use the fresh vegetables to scoop up the hummus and enjoy!

Nutrition Values (per serving, with hummus):

- - Calories: 180 kcal

- - Protein: 6g

- - Fiber: 6g

Note: This hummus and veggie snack platter is a nutritious and satisfying option for seniors with fatty liver disease. Hummus provides protein and healthy fats, while the colorful array of vegetables offers vitamins, minerals, and fiber, making it a well-balanced snack.

Recipe 31: Almond Butter and Banana Slices

Prep Time: 5 minutes - Number of Servings: 2

Ingredients:

- 2 medium ripe bananas, sliced
- 4 tablespoons almond butter (or your preferred nut butter)
- 1 tablespoon chia seeds (optional)
- 1/2 teaspoon ground cinnamon (optional)

Assembly Instructions:

1. Slice the ripe bananas into rounds.
2. Spread almond butter (or your preferred nut butter) on half of the banana slices.
3. Top the almond butter-covered slices with the remaining banana slices to create little banana "sandwiches."
4. If desired, sprinkle chia seeds and a pinch of ground cinnamon over the top for added flavor and texture.
5. Serve immediately for a quick and nutritious snack.

Nutrition Values (per serving, with chia seeds and cinnamon):

- - Calories: 240 kcal
- - Protein: 5g
- - Fiber: 7g

Note: These almond butter and banana slices are a satisfying and energy-boosting snack for seniors with fatty liver disease. Bananas provide potassium and fiber, while almond butter offers healthy fats and a touch of protein.

Recipe 32: Cottage Cheese and Pineapple Delight

Prep Time: 5 minutes - Number of Servings: 2

Ingredients:

- 1 cup low-fat cottage cheese
- 1 cup fresh pineapple chunks (or canned pineapple in natural juice)
- 1/4 cup unsweetened shredded coconut
- 1 tablespoon honey (optional)

Assembly Instructions:

1. In two serving bowls, divide the low-fat cottage cheese evenly.
2. Top the cottage cheese with fresh pineapple chunks.
3. Sprinkle unsweetened shredded coconut over the pineapple.
4. If desired, drizzle honey over the top for a touch of sweetness.
5. Serve immediately for a creamy and tropical-flavored snack.

Nutrition Values (per serving, with honey):

- - Calories: 210 kcal
- - Protein: 15g
- - Fiber: 2g

Note: This cottage cheese and pineapple delight is a creamy and protein-rich snack that's both refreshing and satisfying. Pineapple adds natural sweetness, while cottage cheese provides protein, making it a nutritious choice for liver health.

Recipe 33: Avocado and Tomato Toast

Prep Time: 10 minutes - Number of Servings: 2

Ingredients:

- 2 slices whole grain bread (choose a low-sodium option)
- 1 ripe avocado, peeled and sliced
- 1 medium tomato, sliced
- 1/2 lemon
- Salt and pepper to taste
- Red pepper flakes for garnish (optional)

Assembly Instructions:

1. Toast the slices of whole-grain bread until they are golden brown.
2. While the toast is still warm, divide the ripe avocado slices and place them evenly on each slice.
3. Top the avocado with slices of fresh tomato.
4. Squeeze fresh lemon juice over the avocado and tomato.
5. Season with salt and pepper to taste.
6. If desired, sprinkle red pepper flakes for a hint of spice.
7. Serve immediately for a tasty and heart-healthy snack.

Nutrition Values (per serving):

- - Calories: 200 kcal
- - Protein: 4g
- - Fiber: 7g

Note: This avocado and tomato toast is a satisfying and nutrient-rich snack that's packed with healthy fats, fiber, and vitamins. It's a delicious way to enjoy the creamy goodness of avocado and the freshness of tomatoes.

Recipe 34: Oatmeal Energy Bites

Prep Time: 15 minutes - Chilling Time: 30 minutes - Number of Servings: 12 bites

Ingredients:

- 1 cup old-fashioned oats
- 1/2 cup almond butter (or your preferred nut butter)
- 1/3 cup honey
- 1/4 cup ground flaxseed
- 1/4 cup unsweetened shredded coconut
- 1/4 cup mini chocolate chips (optional)
- 1 teaspoon vanilla extract
- Pinch of salt

Instructions:

1. In a mixing bowl, combine the old-fashioned oats, almond butter, honey, ground flaxseed, unsweetened shredded coconut, mini chocolate chips (if using), vanilla extract, and a pinch of salt.

2. Stir until all the ingredients are well combined.

3. Refrigerate the mixture for about 30 minutes to make it easier to handle.

4. After chilling, use your hands to scoop out portions of the mixture and roll them into bite-sized balls.

5. Place the oatmeal energy bites on a baking sheet lined with parchment paper.

6. Refrigerate for an additional 30 minutes to set.

7. Once firm, transfer the energy bites to an airtight container and store them in the refrigerator until ready to enjoy.

Nutrition Values (per energy bite, without chocolate chips):

- - Calories: 110 kcal
- - Protein: 3g
- - Fiber: 2g

Note: These oatmeal energy bites are a wholesome and energy-boosting snack for seniors with fatty liver disease. They are packed with fiber and healthy fats, making them a satisfying choice for on-the-go nutrition.

Recipe 35: Sliced Apple with Almond Butter

Prep Time: 5 minutes - Number of Servings: 2

Ingredients:

- 1 large apple, thinly sliced
- 4 tablespoons almond butter (or your preferred nut butter)
- Ground cinnamon for garnish (optional)

Assembly Instructions:

1. Wash the apple and thinly slice it into rounds or wedges.
2. Serve the sliced apple with almond butter for dipping.
3. If desired, sprinkle a pinch of ground cinnamon over the apple slices for extra flavor.
4. Enjoy immediately for a crisp and satisfying snack.

Nutrition Values (per serving):

- - Calories: 220 kcal
- - Protein: 6g
- - Fiber: 7g

Note: This sliced apple with almond butter is a classic and nutritious snack that provides a balance of natural sweetness from the apple and healthy fats from the almond butter. It's a quick and easy option for seniors with fatty liver disease.

Chapter 11 – Desserts

Get ready for the conclusion of our ***Fatty Liver Diet Cookbook for Seniors Over 50,*** focusing on a treat. Desserts are designed with the dietary needs of seniors managing fatty liver disease in mind.

When it comes to liver health, desserts don't have to be off-limits. In this chapter, we bring you a selection of seven dessert recipes that are not only tasty but also friendly to your liver. These desserts aim to satisfy your cravings while still aligning with your goals.

We understand the importance of balance when it comes to indulging in sweets. Our recipes are carefully crafted to minimize added sugars and unhealthy fats while maximizing flavor and nutritional value. By incorporating ingredients like fruits, nuts, and whole grains, these desserts offer both taste and health benefits.

Treat yourself guilt-free with options like fruits or yogurt-based parfaits. Each dessert is customized to provide nutrients such as fiber, vitamins, and antioxidants that contribute to your well-being.

Join us on this journey as we demonstrate that enjoying desserts can be part of your liver lifestyle. Desserts can serve as both a reward and a way to nourish your body – let us show you how! Let us explore some dessert recipes that demonstrate how you can enjoy your treats while also considering the health of your liver.

Recipe 36: Baked Apples with Cinnamon and Walnuts

Prep Time: 10 minutes - Cooking Time: 30 minutes - Number of Servings: 2

Ingredients:

- 2 medium apples (e.g., Granny Smith or Honeycrisp)
- 2 tablespoons chopped walnuts
- 1 tablespoon honey or maple syrup
- 1/2 teaspoon ground cinnamon
- 1/4 teaspoon nutmeg (optional)
- 1/4 cup water
- Greek yogurt or low-fat vanilla ice cream for serving (optional)

Cooking Instructions:

1. Preheat your oven to 375°F (190°C).
2. Wash and core the apples, removing the seeds and creating a well in the center.
3. In a small bowl, mix together the chopped walnuts, honey or maple syrup, ground cinnamon, and nutmeg (if using).
4. Stuff each apple with half of the walnut mixture.
5. Place the stuffed apples in a baking dish and pour water into the dish.
6. Cover the dish with foil and bake in the preheated oven for about 25-30 minutes or until the apples are tender and easily pierced with a fork.
7. Remove the foil and bake for an additional 5 minutes to lightly brown the tops.
8. Serve the baked apples with a dollop of Greek yogurt or a scoop of low-fat vanilla ice cream if desired.

Nutrition Values (per serving, without yogurt or ice cream):

- - Calories: 180 kcal
- - Protein: 2g
- - Fiber: 5g

Note: These baked apples with cinnamon and walnuts are a wholesome and naturally sweet dessert option for seniors with fatty liver disease. They provide fiber and antioxidants while satisfying your sweet cravings.

Recipe 37: Chia Seed Pudding with Mixed Berries

Prep Time: 5 minutes (plus chilling time) - Number of Servings: 2

Ingredients:

- 1/4 cup chia seeds
- 1 cup unsweetened almond milk (or your preferred milk)
- 1 tablespoon honey or maple syrup
- 1/2 teaspoon vanilla extract
- 1 cup mixed berries (e.g., strawberries, blueberries, raspberries)
- Fresh mint leaves for garnish (optional)

Instructions:

1. In a bowl, combine chia seeds, unsweetened almond milk, honey or maple syrup, and vanilla extract. Stir well to combine.

2. Cover the bowl and refrigerate for at least 2 hours or overnight to allow the chia seeds to absorb the liquid and create a pudding-like consistency.

3. Before serving, give the chia pudding a good stir to ensure it's well-mixed.

4. Divide the chia pudding into serving glasses or bowls.

5. Top with mixed berries and garnish with fresh mint leaves if desired.

6. Serve chilled as a delightful and nutritious dessert.

Nutrition Values (per serving):

- - Calories: 160 kcal
- - Protein: 4g
- - Fiber: 10g

Note: This chia seed pudding with mixed berries is a creamy and satisfying dessert that's rich in fiber and antioxidants. Chia seeds are packed with essential nutrients, making this a perfect choice for seniors with fatty liver disease.

Recipe 38: Grilled Peaches with Honey and Cinnamon

Prep Time: 5 minutes - Cooking Time: 5 minutes - Number of Servings: 2

Ingredients:

- 2 ripe peaches, halved and pitted
- 1 tablespoon honey
- 1/2 teaspoon ground cinnamon
- Greek yogurt or low-fat vanilla ice cream for serving (optional)

Cooking Instructions:

1. Preheat your grill to medium-high heat.
2. While the grill is heating, drizzle honey over the cut sides of the peach halves and sprinkle them with ground cinnamon.
3. Place the peaches on the grill cut side down.
4. Grill for about 2-3 minutes on each side or until the peaches are tender and have grill marks.
5. Remove the grilled peaches from the grill and let them cool slightly.
6. Serve the grilled peaches with a dollop of Greek yogurt or a scoop of low-fat vanilla ice cream if desired.

Nutrition Values (per serving, without yogurt or ice cream):

- - Calories: 70 kcal
- - Protein: 1g
- - Fiber: 2g

Note: These grilled peaches with honey and cinnamon are a delightful and naturally sweet dessert option for seniors with fatty liver disease. Grilling enhances the peach's flavor, and the honey-cinnamon drizzle adds a touch of warmth and sweetness.

Recipe 39: Berry and Nut Parfait

Prep Time: 10 minutes - Number of Servings: 2

Ingredients:

- 1 cup low-fat Greek yogurt
- 1 cup mixed berries (e.g., strawberries, blueberries, raspberries)
- 2 tablespoons chopped almonds or walnuts
- 1 tablespoon honey or maple syrup
- 1/2 teaspoon vanilla extract

Assembly Instructions:

1. In two serving glasses or bowls, start by adding a layer of low-fat Greek yogurt.
2. Add a layer of mixed berries on top of the yogurt.
3. Sprinkle chopped almonds or walnuts over the berries.
4. Drizzle honey or maple syrup evenly over the parfait.
5. Add a splash of vanilla extract for extra flavor.
6. Repeat the layers if desired.
7. Serve immediately as a creamy and satisfying dessert.

Nutrition Values (per serving):

- - Calories: 250 kcal
- - Protein: 15g
- - Fiber: 5g

Note: This berry and nut parfait is a protein-rich and antioxidant-packed dessert that's perfect for seniors with fatty liver disease. It provides a delightful combination of creamy yogurt, fresh berries, and crunchy nuts.

Recipe 40: Banana and Dark Chocolate Bites

Prep Time: 10 minutes - Freezing Time: 2 hours - Number of Servings: 2

Ingredients:

- 1 large banana, sliced into rounds
- 2 tablespoons dark chocolate chips (70% cocoa or higher)
- 1 tablespoon unsweetened shredded coconut
- 1/4 teaspoon vanilla extract
- Pinch of sea salt

Assembly Instructions:

1. Line a tray or plate with parchment paper.

2. In a microwave-safe bowl, heat the dark chocolate chips in 20-second intervals, stirring between each interval, until they are fully melted and smooth.

3. Stir in the vanilla extract and a pinch of sea salt into the melted chocolate.

4. Dip each banana slice halfway into the melted chocolate and place it on the parchment paper.

5. Sprinkle unsweetened shredded coconut over the chocolate-covered banana slices.

6. Transfer the tray or plate to the freezer and freeze for at least 2 hours or until the chocolate is firm.

7. Once frozen, remove the banana and dark chocolate bites from the freezer and serve as a delightful and satisfying dessert.

Nutrition Values (per serving):

- - Calories: 120 kcal
- - Protein: 1g
- - Fiber: 2g

Note: These banana and dark chocolate bites are a delightful and portion-controlled dessert option for seniors with fatty liver disease. The combination of sweet banana, rich dark chocolate, and a hint of coconut creates a satisfying treat.

Recipe 41: Baked Pears with Cinnamon and Almonds

Prep Time: 10 minutes - Cooking Time: 30 minutes - Number of Servings: 2

Ingredients:

- 2 ripe pears, halved and cored
- 2 tablespoons chopped almonds
- 1 tablespoon honey
- 1/2 teaspoon ground cinnamon
- 1/4 teaspoon vanilla extract
- Greek yogurt or low-fat vanilla ice cream for serving (optional)

Cooking Instructions:

1. Preheat your oven to 375°F (190°C).
2. In a small bowl, combine chopped almonds, honey, ground cinnamon, and vanilla extract. Stir to create a sticky almond topping.
3. Place the pear halves, cut side up, on a baking sheet or in a baking dish.
4. Spoon the almond mixture evenly over the pear halves.
5. Cover the baking sheet or dish with foil and bake in the preheated oven for about 20-25 minutes or until the pears are tender.
6. Remove the foil and bake for an additional 5 minutes to lightly brown the almonds.
7. Serve the baked pears with a dollop of Greek yogurt or a scoop of low-fat vanilla ice cream if desired.

Nutrition Values (per serving, without yogurt or ice cream):

- - Calories: 160 kcal
- - Protein: 2g
- - Fiber: 5g

Note: These baked pears with cinnamon and almonds are a warm and comforting dessert option for seniors with fatty liver disease. The natural sweetness of pears pairs beautifully with the honey-cinnamon almond topping.

Recipe 42: Mixed Berry Frozen Yogurt

Prep Time: 10 minutes (plus freezing time) - Number of Servings: 2

Ingredients:

- 1 cup mixed berries (e.g., strawberries, blueberries, raspberries), frozen
- 1 cup low-fat Greek yogurt
- 2 tablespoons honey or maple syrup
- 1/2 teaspoon vanilla extract
- Fresh mint leaves for garnish (optional)

Instructions:

1. In a food processor or blender, combine the frozen mixed berries, low-fat Greek yogurt, honey or maple syrup, and vanilla extract.

2. Blend until smooth and creamy, scraping down the sides of the container as needed.

3. Taste and adjust the sweetness by adding more honey or maple syrup if desired.

4. Transfer the mixture to a freezer-safe container and freeze for at least 2-3 hours or until firm.

5. Before serving, allow the frozen yogurt to sit at room temperature for a few minutes to soften slightly.

6. Scoop the mixed berry frozen yogurt into serving bowls or glasses.

7. Garnish with fresh mint leaves if desired.

8. Enjoy this cool and fruity dessert.

Nutrition Values (per serving):

- - Calories: 180 kcal

- - Protein: 10g

- - Fiber: 3g

Note: This mixed berry frozen yogurt is a refreshing and guilt-free dessert option for seniors with fatty liver disease. It's made with wholesome ingredients and provides the sweetness of mixed berries without added sugars.

Chapter 12: A 7-Day Meal Plan

Welcome to the core of our *Fatty Liver Diet Cookbook for Seniors Over 50*. In this chapter, we present a crafted 7-day meal plan specifically designed to support and nurture seniors who are dealing with fatty liver disease.

We understand that adhering to a diet can be quite challenging. It is an essential step in maintaining liver health. This meal plan removes any guesswork when it comes to your nutrition, providing you with a week's worth of balanced and delicious meals that cater to the dietary requirements of individuals managing fatty liver disease.

Each day of this meal plan offers a selection of breakfasts, lunches, and courses accompanied by sides and desserts. We have chosen recipes that prioritize liver health while ensuring that your meals remain satisfying and bursting with flavors.

Our aim is to demonstrate that eating for liver health can be a sustainable journey. The recipes included in this meal plan incorporate ingredients known for their friendliness towards the liver, such as proteins, whole grains, fruits, vegetables, and healthy fats. By following this plan, you can take strides towards managing your fatty liver while relishing the joys of food.

Whether you are new to managing fatty liver disease or seeking inspiration, this meal plan serves as your guide toward a well-rounded and nourishing diet.

Join us on a 7-day exploration where we indulge in exciting flavors while nurturing our taste buds and promoting liver health. Let's kickstart this week's wellness adventure, savoring each meal along the way.

Day 1:

Breakfast:

- Oatmeal with Berries and Almonds
   - Prep Time: 5 minutes
   - Number of Servings: 1

Lunch:

- Spinach and Quinoa Salad with Lemon Vinaigrette
   - Prep Time: 15 minutes
   - Number of Servings: 2

Main Course with Side:

- Baked Salmon with Roasted Vegetables
   - Prep Time: 15 minutes
   - Cooking Time: 25 minutes
   - Number of Servings: 2
- Steamed Asparagus with Garlic and Lemon
   - Prep Time: 10 minutes
   - Cooking Time: 5 minutes
   - Number of Servings: 2

Dessert:

- Baked Apples with Cinnamon and Walnuts
   - Prep Time: 10 minutes
   - Cooking Time: 30 minutes
   - Number of Servings: 2

Day 2:

Breakfast:

- Scrambled Eggs with Spinach and Tomato
  - Prep Time: 10 minutes
  - Number of Servings: 1

Lunch:

- Quinoa and Black Bean Salad with Avocado Dressing
  - Prep Time: 15 minutes
  - Number of Servings: 2

Main Course with Side:

- Grilled Chicken Breast with Brown Rice
  - Prep Time: 10 minutes
  - Cooking Time: 20 minutes
  - Number of Servings: 2
- Roasted Brussels Sprouts with Balsamic Glaze
  - Prep Time: 10 minutes
  - Cooking Time: 25 minutes
  - Number of Servings: 2

Dessert:

- Chia Seed Pudding with Mixed Berries
  - Prep Time: 5 minutes (plus chilling time)
  - Number of Servings: 2

Day 3:

Breakfast:

- Greek Yogurt Parfait with Honey and Nuts
  - Prep Time: 5 minutes
  - Number of Servings: 1

Lunch:

- Lentil Soup with Spinach and Carrots
  - Prep Time: 15 minutes
  - Cooking Time: 30 minutes
  - Number of Servings: 2

Main Course with Side:

- Baked Tilapia with Quinoa Pilaf
  - Prep Time: 15 minutes
  - Cooking Time: 25 minutes
  - Number of Servings: 2
- Sautéed Green Beans with Almonds and Lemon
  - Prep Time: 10 minutes
  - Cooking Time: 10 minutes
  - Number of Servings: 2

Dessert:

- Grilled Peaches with Honey and Cinnamon
  - Prep Time: 5 minutes
  - Cooking Time: 5 minutes
  - Number of Servings: 2

Day 4:

Breakfast:

- Berry and Spinach Smoothie
  - Prep Time: 5 minutes
  - Number of Servings: 1

Lunch:

- Turkey and Vegetable Wrap
  - Prep Time: 10 minutes
  - Number of Servings: 2

Main Course with Side:

- Recipe Grilled Shrimp with Brown Rice and Broccoli
  - Prep Time: 15 minutes
  - Cooking Time: 15 minutes
  - Number of Servings: 2
- Recipe 25: Mashed Cauliflower with Garlic and Chives
  - Prep Time: 10 minutes
  - Cooking Time: 15 minutes
  - Number of Servings: 2

Dessert:

- Berry and Nut Parfait
  - Prep Time: 10 minutes
  - Number of Servings: 2

Day 5:

Breakfast:

- Whole-grain pancakes with Fresh Fruit
  - Prep Time: 15 minutes
  - Number of Servings: 1

Lunch:

- Chickpea and Vegetable Salad with Lemon-Tahini Dressing
  - Prep Time: 15 minutes
  - Number of Servings: 2

Main Course with Side:

- Baked Chicken Thighs with Sweet Potato Mash
  - Prep Time: 15 minutes
  - Cooking Time: 40 minutes
  - Number of Servings: 2
- Sautéed Spinach with Garlic and Pine Nuts
  - Prep Time: 10 minutes
  - Cooking Time: 10 minutes
  - Number of Servings: 2

Dessert:

- Banana and Dark Chocolate Bites
  - Prep Time: 10 minutes
  - Freezing Time: 2 hours
  - Number of Servings: 2

Day 6:

Breakfast:

- Greek Yogurt and Berry Parfait
  - Prep Time: 5 minutes
  - Number of Servings: 1

Lunch:

- Tuna Salad with Mixed Greens
  - Prep Time: 10 minutes
  - Number of Servings: 2

Main Course with Side:

- Stir-fried tofu with Brown Rice and Broccoli
  - Prep Time: 15 minutes
  - Cooking Time: 15 minutes
  - Number of Servings: 2
- Roasted Carrots with Rosemary and Thyme
  - Prep Time: 10 minutes
  - Cooking Time: 25 minutes
  - Number of Servings: 2

Dessert:

- Baked Pears with Cinnamon and Almonds
  - Prep Time: 10 minutes
  - Cooking Time: 30 minutes
  - Number of Servings: 2

Day 7:

Breakfast:

- Overnight Chia Pudding with Berries
  - Prep Time: 5 minutes (plus chilling time)
  - Number of Servings: 1

Lunch:

- Vegetable and Lentil Soup
  - Prep Time: 15 minutes
  - Cooking Time: 30 minutes
  - Number of Servings: 2

Main Course with Side:

- Steamed Asparagus with Garlic and Lemon
  - Prep Time: 10 minutes
  - Cooking Time: 5 minutes
  - Number of Servings: 2
- Quinoa with Roasted Vegetables
  - Prep Time: 15 minutes
  - Cooking Time: 30 minutes
  - Number of Servings: 2

Dessert:

- Mixed Berry Frozen Yogurt
  - Prep Time: 10 minutes (plus freezing time)
  - Number of Servings: 2

Chapter 13: Questions and Answers About Fatty Liver

Q1: What are the three indications of a fatty liver?

A1: Fatigue, discomfort or fullness in the abdomen, and unexplained weight loss are three common signs that may indicate a fatty liver.

Q2: How can I improve my fatty liver condition?

A2: Lifestyle changes play a role in improving the health of your fatty liver. These changes include maintaining a weight, adopting a diet, engaging in regular physical activity, limiting alcohol consumption, effectively managing underlying conditions such as diabetes, and avoiding foods high in added sugars and unhealthy fats.

Q3: Can fatty liver be reversed?

A3: With lifestyle modifications, a fatty liver can show improvement or even reverse. However, the outcome may vary depending on the severity of the condition and its underlying causes. It is important to work with healthcare professionals to monitor and manage this condition.

Q4: Is fatty liver considered an issue?

A4: Fatty liver is indeed a health concern that can lead to severe liver complications if left untreated. It has the potential to progress into conditions such as alcoholic steatohepatitis (NASH) cirrhosis or even develop into liver cancer. Early diagnosis, along with lifestyle adjustments, are critical.

Q5: Which foods should be avoided if one has been diagnosed with fatty liver?

A5: If you have a fatty liver, it is recommended to limit or avoid foods high in added sugars, saturated fats, and trans fats. These include drinks, processed foods, fried foods, and excessive consumption of processed meats.

Q6: How long does it take to reverse a fatty liver?

A6: The time it takes to reverse a fatty liver can vary from person to person. It depends on factors such as the severity of the condition, how well lifestyle changes are followed, and individual health. Improvement may be observed within months and may take up to a year or even longer.

Q7: What beverages can I consume to support liver detoxification?

A7: To promote liver health, it is beneficial to drink an amount of water along with tea and herbal teas like dandelion or milk thistle. These beverages may assist in natural detoxification processes within the liver.

Q8: Can apple cider vinegar help cleanse the liver?

A8: While there is evidence specifically supporting apple cider vinegar's ability to directly "cleanse" the liver, some individuals believe that consuming it in moderation can contribute to overall digestive health.

Q9: What is the medication for treating fatty liver?

A9: Currently, there are no specific medications approved for treating fatty liver disease. Treatment primarily focuses on making changes to your lifestyle, managing your weight, and addressing any conditions like diabetes or high cholesterol. It is recommended to consult with a healthcare professional for guidance.

Q10: Can I eat eggs if I have liver?

A10: Including eggs in a balanced diet is acceptable for someone with fatty liver. They provide an amount of protein and essential nutrients. However, it is important to consume them in moderation and prepare them in a way such as boiling, poaching, or frying.

Q11: What is the main food that causes liver?

A11: One of the leading culprits associated with fatty liver is beverages, those that contain high fructose corn syrup. Consuming amounts of added sugars has been linked to the development and progression of fatty liver disease.

Q12: What are some signs that indicate a damaged liver?

A12: There are warning signs that may indicate damage to the liver, including jaundice (yellowing of the skin and eyes), abdominal pain or swelling, dark urine, and unusual fatigue.

Q13: What kind of pain do you experience with a fatty liver?

A13: Discomfort or a sense of fullness in the abdomen can commonly be experienced by individuals with fatty liver.

Q14: What is the initial stage of fatty liver?

A14: The initial phase of fatty liver disease is typically referred to as fatty liver or steatosis. In this stage, it accumulates in the liver cells without inflammation or scarring.

Q15: What is the amount of weight loss required to reverse fatty liver?

A15: The weight loss needed to reverse fatty liver varies from person to person. It is often recommended to start with a sustained weight loss of 5% to 10% of body weight in order to improve liver health.

CAUTION: Please note that these responses offer information and are not meant to replace personalized advice. For guidance regarding your health and condition, it is important to consult with a healthcare provider.

About The Author

Samantha Bax, an advocate of vegan, friendly, and renal-conscious cuisine, found her true calling in the heart of a bustling city. Then, starting her journey in a professional kitchen, it all began in her grandmother's cozy home, where she first learned the value of wholesome and nutritious eating.

When Samantha was diagnosed with diabetes in her twenties, her life took a turn. This pivotal moment fueled her dedication to health and wellness, ultimately leading her to become a certified nutritionist. However, fate had a plan for Samantha when a close family member was diagnosed with kidney disease. This significant event merged her two passions for food and well-being, inspiring her to create a niche that caters to both diabetic and renal diets.

Course Samantha encountered challenges along the way. Balancing health requirements with flavors proved to be complex. However, she remained steadfast in refusing to compromise taste for the sake of health. To overcome this hurdle, Samantha embarked on a culinary adventure where she drew inspiration from kitchens across the Mediterranean region, spice markets in Asia, and farms throughout Central America.

In **"Fatty Liver Cookbook for Seniors Over 50: Low Carb Recipes And Cleansing Methods To Combat Fatty Liver And Fibrosis."** Samantha Bax masterfully combines her story with a collection of mouth-watering recipes. She firmly believes that while food is essential for survival, it should also be cherished as a celebration of life and well-being.

In this book, her goal is to offer readers a collection of recipes that cater to their needs while also providing an enjoyable culinary experience.

Outside of writing and culinary experimentation, Samantha finds joy in the art of photography. She captures the essence of both cityscapes and peaceful natural landscapes. Additionally, she leads workshops and seminars where she guides individuals in making food choices that don't compromise on taste.

To join our Newsletter and receive advance notification of new publications, subscribe to the Newsletter for FREE today at:

www.prosebooks.us/subscribe